THE ULTIMATE COOKBOOK

For Acid Reflux Relief

Delicious and Effortless Recipes for Easy Acid Reflux Control

Joan R. Cottrell

SCAN THE QR CODE FOR MORE COOKBOOKS BY THE AUTHOR

Contents

Always prioritize self-care and be gentle with yourself. Small changes to your diet and lifestyle can have a big impact.

Sarah's story

Nothing seemed to help Sarah when she had acid reflux, despite her trying everything to manage it, including prescription and over-the-counter medications. It wasn't until she spoke with her friend Mary—who also suffered from acid reflux—that she began to regain hope. Mary shared with her some new recipes she had discovered that were made especially for those who suffer from acid reflux. Despite her initial skepticism, Sarah chose to give it a shot by attempting the recipes in this cookbook.

Sarah started by making breakfast, lunch, and dinner according to the cookbook's instructions. To have more control over the ingredients she was consuming, she also began preparing more meals at home. In just a few weeks, Sarah saw a significant improvement. Her symptoms of acid reflux had significantly decreased, and she could now enjoy her food without worrying about a flare-up.

She was overjoyed to have discovered the recipes, as they had allowed her to manage her acid reflux and resume a regular life.

You can find a compilation of tasty and easy recipes created especially for those who suffer from acid reflux in *"The Ultimate Cookbook for Acid Reflux Relief: Delicious and Effortless Recipes for Easy Acid Reflux Control."* The recipes are simple to follow and make use of well-known reflux-friendly ingredients.

A section on the fundamentals of acid reflux, including what it is, what causes it, and how to treat it, is also included in the cookbook. You can use this information to better understand your health and make decisions that will benefit your well-being.

I strongly recommend that you try the recipes in this cookbook if you are having trouble managing your acid reflux. Sarah and many others have benefited from their assistance in getting their symptoms under control. I hope that the recipes in this cookbook can assist you as well.

Let's get cooking!

Chapter 1:
What Exactly Is Acid Reflux?

Acid reflux occurs when stomach acid backs up into the esophagus, which connects the mouth to the stomach. This can result in heartburn, a burning sensation in the chest, as well as other symptoms such as a sour taste in the mouth, difficulty swallowing, and a cough.

Causes of Acid Reflux

The lower esophageal sphincter (LES) is a muscle at the bottom of the esophagus that normally opens to allow food into the stomach and then closes tightly.

The LES weakens or relaxes too frequently in acid reflux patients, allowing stomach acid to back up into the esophagus.

Acid reflux can be caused by a variety of factors, including:

- Eating a lot of food
- Consuming certain foods and beverages, such as fatty or spicy foods, caffeine, and alcoholic beverages
- Sleeping too soon after eating
- Obesity is a problem.
- Maternity
- Cigarette smoking
- Specific medications

Quick Tips on How to Deal With Acid Reflux
You can manage acid reflux by doing the following things:

- Avoid foods and beverages that make your symptoms worse.
- Consume smaller, more frequent meals.
- If you are overweight or obese, you should lose weight.
- Avoid lying down immediately after eating.
- Raise the head of your bed 6-8 inches.
- Use over-the-counter or prescription drugs

Cooking Suggestions for Acid Reflux

If you have acid reflux, you can reduce your symptoms by doing the following while cooking:

- Refrain from using butter or fatty oils like olive or vegetable oil. Use nonfat cooking sprays or water instead.
- Stay away from acidic ingredients like tomatoes, citrus juices, and vinegar.
- To avoid indigestion, thoroughly cook meats and vegetables.
- Limit your intake of large meals. Eat smaller, more frequent meals instead.
- Avoid lying down immediately after eating.

Chapter 2:
Breakfast

Oatmeal with Berries and Nuts

Total Time: 15 Minutes
Servings: 2 people

Ingredients:

- 3/4 cup organic old-fashioned oats
- 1.5 cups water
- 2 tablespoons ground flaxseeds
- 1 tablespoon chia seeds
- 1/4 teaspoon salt
- 1 cup organic berries (I frequently use frozen)
- 1 tablespoon walnuts or mixed nuts

Directions:

1. 1 1/2 cups water, oatmeal, ground flax, chia seeds, and salt should be brought to a boil.
2. Reduce the heat to low and continue to cook for 7-10 minutes, or until the water has evaporated and the oatmeal is soft.
3. Berries should be cut into bite-sized pieces.
4. With soy yogurt or nut milk, top the oatmeal with the berries and nuts.

Fruit And Yogurt Parfait with Granola

Total Time: 5 minutes
Servings: 1 large parfait

Ingredients:

- 1/2 cup plain Greek yogurt
- 1/2 cup granola (make your own almond pecan granola or coconut maple walnut granola)
- 1/2 cup fruit
- Optional: honey

Directions:

1. Pour 1/4 cup yogurt into the bottom of a tall rounded glass. Spread 1/4 cup granola on top and smooth. Smooth out 1/4 cup of fruit on top.
2. Continue with the remaining ingredients.
3. Drizzle honey on top for extra sweetness.

Egg White Omelet with Spinach and Cheese

Total Time: 5 minutes total
Servings:1

Ingredients:

- Three large egg whites
- Coarse salt and freshly ground pepper
- 1 tablespoon olive oil
- 1 cup baby spinach, packed
- 1/4 cup (1%) low-fat cottage cheese
- 2 tbsp. grated Parmesan

Directions:

1. Whisk together egg whites and 1 tablespoon water in a medium mixing bowl; season with salt and pepper and set aside.
2. Heat the oil in a medium nonstick skillet over medium-high heat. Season the spinach with salt and pepper and cook for 1 minute, or until wilted and tender. Cook until nearly set, 1 to 2 minutes, using a flexible heatproof spatula to pull the sides of the omelet toward the center as uncooked egg whites run underneath.
3. Dollop cottage cheese over omelet, top with Parmesan, and season with salt and pepper. Gently slide the omelet onto a serving plate, folding it over on itself by slightly tilting the skillet.

....

Continue to seek medical advice, investigate different options,
and rely on the support of friends and family.

....

Chapter 3:
Snacks and Side Dishes

Roasted Vegetables

Total time:1 hour 5 minutes
serves 10

Ingredients:

- 2 red bell peppers
- 1 onion, red
- 1 pound butternut squash
- 6 young leeks
- 4 courgettes, preferably of different colors
- one aubergine
- 2 tomato
- 6 garlic cloves
- 1 tbsp. coriander seeds
- a pinch of sea salt
- freshly milled black pepper
- 1 sprig of fresh rosemary
- 1 sprig of fresh thyme
- extra virgin olive oil

Directions:

To prepare your vegetables:

1. Preheat the oven to 200°C/400°F/gas 6 and set aside.
   After halving and deseeding the pepper, cut each half
   into four pieces.
2. Peel and cut the red onion into 8 wedges. Cut the
   squash in half carefully, then scoop out and discard the
   seeds.
3. Each half should be cut into 2cm chunks. Baby leeks
   should be washed and trimmed. Cut the courgettes in
   half lengthwise, then slice them into 2cm chunks.
4. Remove the top and tail of the aubergine and cut it into
   quarters, then into 2cm chunks. Cut the tomatoes into
   quarters. Keep the garlic cloves in their skins, but
   squash them with the heel of your hand.
5. Place all of the vegetables in an extra-large roasting
   tray or two smaller ones. In a pestle and mortar, crush
   the coriander seeds, then sprinkle over the vegetables
   with a generous pinch of salt and pepper.
6. The rosemary leaves should be picked and roughly
   chopped. Gather the thyme leaves. Scatter the herbs
   over the vegetables. Drizzle olive oil over everything
   and toss to coat.

How to Cook and Serve Vegetables:

1. Cook your vegetables in a hot oven for 50 minutes, or
   until soft, golden, and cooked through.
2. Toss with pasta or couscous for a quick veggie meal,
   or serve with anything from roast chicken to grilled
   meats or fish.

Mashed Potatoes

Total Time: 45 minutes

10 to 12 servings

Ingredients:

- 5 pounds potatoes (I use half Yukon Gold and half Russet).
- 2 large garlic cloves, minced
- coarse sea salt
- 6 tbsp. melted butter
- 1-quart whole milk
- 4 ounces room temperature cream cheese

Toppings:

- fresh chives or green onions, chopped
- freshly ground black pepper

Directions:

1. Peel or leave the skins on your potatoes. Then, cut them into evenly sized chunks about an inch thick and place them in a large stockpot filled with cold water.
2. Once you've cut all of your potatoes, fill the pan with cold water until the water line is about 1 inch above the potatoes. In a small bowl, combine the garlic and 1 tablespoon of sea salt.
3. Then, increase the heat to high and continue to cook until the water comes to a boil. Reduce heat to medium-high (or whatever temperature is required to keep the boil going) and cook for 10-12 minutes, or

until a knife inserted into the center of a potato goes in easily and almost without resistance. Drain all of the water carefully.

4. While the potatoes are boiling, combine the butter, milk, and an additional 2 teaspoons of sea salt in a small saucepan or microwave until the butter is just melted. (You don't want to boil the milk.) Set aside until ready to use.

5. After draining the water, return the potatoes to the hot stockpot, replace them on the hot burner, and reduce the heat to low.

6. Holding the stockpot handles with two oven mitts, gently shake it on the burner for about 1 minute to help cook off some of the remaining steam within the potatoes.

7. Remove the stockpot from the heat and place it on a flat, heat-resistant surface.

8. Mash the potatoes to the desired consistency with your preferred type of potato masher.

9. Then, pour half of the melted butter mixture over the potatoes, folding it in with a wooden spoon or spatula until the potatoes have absorbed the liquid.

10. Repeat with the remaining butter and cream cheese, folding in each addition until just combined to avoid over-mixing. (If necessary, add more warm milk to achieve the desired consistency.)

11. Taste the potatoes one last time and season with additional salt if necessary.

12. Then serve warm, garnished with gravy or any additional toppings you desire, and enjoy!

Sweet Potato Fries

Prep:2 mins
Cooking time:20 mins
1 serving

Ingredients:

- 95g sweet potato sliced into fries
- 1 teaspoon rapeseed oil
- 1/4 teaspoon cayenne pepper

Directions:

1. Preheat the oven to 200°C/180°C fan/gas 6.
2. Place 95g sweet potato fries on a baking tray and toss with 1 tablespoon rapeseed oil and 1/4 teaspoon cayenne pepper.
3. Cook for 20 minutes in the oven.

Whole-Wheat Rolls

Preparation Time: 2 hours 30 minutes
Cooking Time: 25 minutes
Total Time: 2 hours 55 minutes
Yield: 24 rolls

Ingredients:

- 2 tbsp active dry yeast* (instant yeast also works)
- 1/2 cup hot water
- 1/2 cup softened butter
- 1 tablespoon honey
- 3 eggs
- 1 cup lukewarm milk or buttermilk
- 4 1/2–5 cups whole wheat flour
- 1 1/2 teaspoon salt

Directions:

1. In a glass measure, dissolve the yeast in 1/2 cup warm water. Place aside.
2. In the bowl of a stand mixer fitted with the paddle attachment, cream the butter and honey. Scrape the sides of the bowl as you mix in the eggs.
3. Combine the yeast mixture with the warmed milk.
4. Mix in 4 1/2 cup flour and the salt until well combined.
5. Switch to the dough hook and knead for 2-3 minutes, or until the dough is no longer tacky, adding a tablespoon or two of flour at a time if necessary. (Do not overdo it.)
6. Allow for one hour in a covered bowl.

7. Turn out onto a floured surface and knead a few times before resting for 3 minutes.
8. Divide the mixture into 24 equal pieces, shape each into a ball, and place in a buttered 13x9-inch baking dish, touching the pieces.
9. Allow to rise for 1 hour, covered.
10. Preheat the oven to 350°F.
11. 20-25 minutes, or until golden brown.

Cornbread

Prep:10 Min
Total:35 Min
Servings:12

Ingredients:

- 3/4 cup medium grind yellow cornmeal
- 1 1/2 cups plain or all-purpose flour
- 1 tablespoon baking powder
- 1/2 cup granulated sugar
- 1/4 teaspoon salt
- 1 cup creamed corn, canned
- 1/2 cup / 125g unsalted melted butter
- 2 lightly whisked eggs
- 3/4 cup milk

Baking

- 1 - 2 tbsp melted butter (for greasing and brushing)

Directions:

1. While making the batter, preheat an oven skillet to 220C / 425F.
2. Combine the Dry Ingredients in a mixing bowl.
3. In a separate mixing bowl, combine the wet ingredients.
4. Pour the wet ingredients into the dry ingredients and stir until combined.
5. Remove the skillet from the oven. Swirl in 1 tablespoon of butter to coat the bottom and halfway up the sides (or use a brush to do this).
6. Pour the batter in and smooth the top.
7. Reduce the oven temperature to 190°C/375°F and bake for 25 to 30 minutes, or until the top is light golden brown and a skewer inserted into the center comes out clean (or the top springs back when poked).
8. Allow to cool in the skillet for 15 minutes before turning out onto a serving platter or cutting board.
9. Best served hot! It can be served directly from the skillet or turned out. Serve with butter and honey to make it extra special!

Salad with Vinaigrette Dressing

Prep/Total Time: 15 min.
5 servings

Ingredients:

- 5 cups salad greens, mixed

- 1 small tomato, peeled and cut into wedges
- 1 cup thinly sliced cucumber
- 1 small red onion, peeled and sliced into rings
- 1/3 cup olive oil
- 2 tablespoons red wine vinegar plus 1 1/2 teaspoons
- 3/4 teaspoon sugar
- 1 tsp. Italian seasoning
- 1/2 tsp lemon juice
- 1 minced garlic clove
- Season with salt and pepper to taste

Directions:

1. Toss the greens, tomato, cucumber, and onion in a salad bowl.
2. Combine the remaining ingredients in a jar with a tight-fitting lid; shake well.
3. Just before serving, drizzle dressing over the salad.

Fruit Salad

Preparation time: 15 minutes
6-8 servings

Ingredients:

- 2 kiwi
- 1 mango
- 150 grams pineapple
- 100g of grapes
- 400g berries (strawberries, raspberries, and blackberries)

- 1 medium orange
- 2 teaspoon honey (optional)

Directions:

1. Use a small serrated knife to cut the fruit. Remove the top and bottom of the kiwi, then stand it up on one of its flat surfaces and cut away the skin as close to the skin as possible.
2. Cut each half in half, following the core through the center, and then into slices. Put one kiwi in a bowl and repeat with the other.
3. Remove the skin from the mango and slice off each cheek, getting as close to the stone as possible. Each piece should be cut into slices.
4. Remove any remaining fruit from the stone by cutting it into long, thin slices. Combine the mango and kiwi.
5. Top and tail the pineapple then cut away the skin in the same manner as the kiwi. By going around the pineapple and removing the dives or eyes two to three at a time, you'll have a spiral pattern weaving around the outside of the fruit.
6. Take a 150g circular slice, quarter it, remove the core, and cut it into chunks. Add to the mixing bowl.
7. Half the grapes and add them to the rest of the fruit, along with the berries; if the strawberries are large, slice or halve them. Peel the orange in the same way that you did the kiwi and pineapple.

8. Holding the orange over the bowl of fruit, carefully cut between the membrane and the fruit to remove the orange segments.
9. The pieces, along with any juice, should fall into the bowl. Squeeze the membrane over the fruit to extract the juice; drizzle with honey if desired.
10. If you have time, combine everything and place it in the fridge to macerate for 30 minutes.

Fruity Yogurt Dip

Preparation Time: 5 minutes
Total Time: 5 minutes
Each dip yields 8-10 servings.

Ingredients:

- 1/2 cup thawed fresh or frozen berries (strawberries or mixed berries)
- 3/4 cup plain Greek yogurt (nonfat, 2%, or 5%)
- Serve with fresh berries, banana slices, apple wedges, graham crackers, and so on.

Directions:

1. Place the berries in a blender and puree until smooth.
2. In a small mixing bowl, combine the berry puree and Greek yogurt until well combined.
3. Serve immediately with graham crackers and fresh fruit. Leftovers can be stored in the refrigerator, covered, for up to a week.

Guacamole

Preparation time: 10 minutes
Total time: 10 minutes
Servings: 4

Ingredients:

- 3 ripe avocados
- 1/2 finely diced small yellow onion
- 2 diced Roma tomatoes
- 3 tbsp fresh cilantro, finely chopped
- 1 jalapeno pepper (seeded and finely diced)
- 2 minced garlic cloves
- 1 lime, freshly squeezed
- 1/2 tsp sea salt

Directions:

1. Cut the avocados in half, scoop out the pit, and place in a mixing bowl.
2. With a fork, mash the avocado until it's as chunky or smooth as you like.
3. Combine the remaining ingredients in a mixing bowl. Taste it and adjust with more salt or lime juice as needed.
4. Guacamole should be served with tortilla chips.

Trail Mix

Preparation Time: 5 minutes
Time allotted: 5 minutes
Yield: 4–5 cups

Ingredient:

- 1 1/2 cups raw nuts, such as almonds, pecans, cashews, peanuts, and so on.
- 1 cup raw seeds, such as sunflower seeds or pumpkin seeds
- 1 cup dried fruit, unsweetened and unsulphured
- Snacks (amounts vary), such as 1/2 cup chopped dark chocolate, 1 cup popped popcorn, 1 cup pretzels, and so on.
- Spices, such as 1/4 teaspoon sea salt, 1/2 teaspoon cinnamon, and a pinch of nutmeg (optional)

Trail Mix Recipe:

- 3/4 cup raw pecans (toasted in the oven for 10 minutes at 350°F)
- 3/4 cup raw cashews (toasted in the oven for 10 minutes at 350°F)
- 1/2 cup uncooked sunflower seeds
- 1/2 cup uncooked pumpkin seeds
- 1/2 cup unsweetened cherries
- 1/2 cup unsweetened raisins
- 1/2 cup 82% dark chocolate, chopped
- 1/4 teaspoon sea salt
- 1/2 teaspoon cinnamon
- nutmeg pinch

Directions:

1. In a large mixing bowl, combine all of the ingredients and thoroughly combine.
2. Place in a ziploc bag or mason jar to keep.
3. Will last up to a month.
4. Optional: To add extra sweetness, coat the mix with 2 tbsp maple syrup, spread it out on a baking sheet, and allow it to dry before bagging.

Chapter 4:
Soups and Salads

Chicken Noodle Soup

Preparation time: 20 minutes
Cooking time: 20 minutes
Total time: 40 minutes
Servings:8

Ingredients:

Soup Ingredients:

- 1/2 teaspoon butter
- 2 ribs of diced celery
- 3-4 large diced carrots
- 1 minced garlic clove
- 10 cup chicken broth or stock
- 1 tsp salt, to taste
- To taste, 1/2 teaspoon freshly ground black pepper
- 1/8 teaspoon dried rosemary (or more as desired)
- 1/8 teaspoon sage dried
- 1/8 teaspoon red pepper flakes, crushed
- 1 batch of homemade egg noodles* or 5 cups dry egg noodles, farfalle, or other small pasta
- 3 cups rotisserie chicken
- 1 teaspoon better than bouillon chicken flavor (or more if necessary) or chicken bouillon granules

Directions:

1. In a large stockpot over medium-high heat, combine the butter, celery, and carrots. Cook for 3 minutes. Cook for another 30 seconds after adding the garlic.
2. Season the broth with rosemary, sage, crushed red pepper, salt (definitely TASTE the broth before adding additional salt), and pepper. As needed, season with a spoonful of "better than bullion" chicken or chicken bouillon cubes or granules.
3. Bring the broth up to a boil. Cook until the noodles are al dente (either uncooked homemade egg noodles or dry store-bought pasta).
4. When using store-bought noodles, take care not to overcook them! Remove from heat when they are just barely tender. When you remove the pot from the heat, the noodles will continue to cook, and you don't want them mushy.
5. Combine the chicken meat from the rotisserie chicken. Taste the broth again and adjust the seasonings if necessary.
6. Refrigerate leftovers in an airtight container for 4-5 days, depending on the freshness of the chicken you use.

Lentil Soup

Ingredients:

- 2 tablespoons olive oil
- 1 chopped onion (white, brown, or yellow)
- 2 minced garlic cloves
- 1 large carrot, chopped (approximately 1 1/4 cup)
- 2 chopped celery ribs (about 1 1/4 cup)
- 2 cups / 400g rinsed dried green or brown lentils (Note 1)
- 400g crushed tomato (14 oz)
- 1.5 liters / 1.5 quarts (6 cups) low sodium vegetable or chicken stock / broth
- 1/2 teaspoon cumin and coriander powder each
- 1/2 teaspoon paprika powder
- 2 bay leaves, dried
- 1 lemon (zest and juice)
- 1/4 teaspoon salt and pepper

To be served:

- Freshly chopped parsley for garnish
- Serve with warm bread

Directions:

1. In a large pot, heat the oil over medium heat. Cook for 2 minutes after adding the garlic and onion.

2. Mix in the celery and carrot. Cook for 7 to 10 minutes, or until the onion is softened and sweet. Don't rush through this step; it's crucial to the soup's flavor base.
3. Except for the lemon and salt, combine the remaining ingredients. Stir.
4. Increase the heat to a simmer. Scoop the scum off the surface and discard (do this again during cooking if necessary). Replace the lid and reduce the heat to medium-low. Simmer for 35-40 minutes, or until the lentils are tender.
5. Take out the bay leaves.
6. Thicken the soup with 2 or 3 quick whizzes of a stick blender (see video below). Alternatively, transfer 2 cups to a blender, allow to cool slightly, then cover with a tea towel and blend before returning to the pot.
7. If you want to change the consistency of the soup, add a splash of water. Season with salt and pepper to taste. Grate over the lemon zest and finish with a squeeze of lemon juice just before serving. If desired, garnish with parsley and serve with warm crusty bread slathered liberally with butter!

Vegetable Soup

Preparation Time: 15 minutes
Cooking Time: 45 minutes
Total Time: 1 hour and 15 minutes
Servings per recipe: 8

Ingredients:

- 2 tablespoons olive oil
- 1 medium chopped yellow onion
- 2 chopped large carrots
- 1 cup celery, chopped
- 28 oz diced canned tomatoes
- 60 oz low-sodium vegetable broth
- 3 medium diced potatoes
- 1 cup chopped green beans
- three bay leaves
- 2 teaspoon salt (or to taste)
- 1 teaspoon ground black pepper
- 1 cup sweet maize, frozen
- 1 cup sweet peas, frozen
- 1/2 cup chopped green onions
- 1/4 cup chopped fresh parsley

Directions:

1. Preheat a large soup pot or Dutch oven over medium heat with 2 tablespoons olive oil. Sauté the onions and carrots for 6-8 minutes, stirring occasionally, until golden.
2. Combine celery, canned tomatoes (with juice), broth, potatoes, green beans, bay leaves, salt, and pepper in a

large mixing bowl. Bring to a boil, then reduce to low heat and cook for 25 minutes.

3. Add corn, sweet peas, green onion, and parsley once the vegetables are tender. Season with salt to taste, and continue to cook for another 5-8 minutes. Remove from the heat and serve hot.

Minestrone Soup

Preparation Time: 15 minutes
Cooking Time: 30 minutes
Serves 4 to 6 people

Ingredients:

- 2 tbsp extra-virgin olive oil
- 1 medium diced yellow onion
- 2 medium carrots, diced
- 2 thinly sliced celery ribs
- 1 teaspoon sea salt, plus additional to taste
- Ground black pepper, freshly ground
- 3 grated garlic cloves
- 1 can diced tomatoes (28 oz.)
- 1 1/2 cups cooked, drained, and rinsed white beans or kidney beans
- 1 cup green beans, chopped
- 4 cups veggie broth
- two bay leaves
- 1 tsp dried oregano
- 1 tsp. dried thyme
- 3/4 cup small elbows, shells, orecchiette

- 1/2 cup fresh parsley, chopped
- A few pinches of red pepper flakes
- Optional grated Parmesan cheese for serving

Directions:

1. In a large pot, heat the oil over medium heat. Cook, stirring occasionally, for 8 minutes, or until the vegetables begin to soften, with the onion, carrots, celery, salt, and several grinds of black pepper.
2. Combine the garlic, tomatoes, beans, green beans, broth, bay leaves, oregano, and thyme in a large mixing bowl. Cook for 20 minutes, covered.
3. Stir in the pasta and cook, uncovered, for 10 minutes, or until the pasta is tender.
4. Season with salt and pepper to taste, and top with parsley, red pepper flakes, and parmesan if desired.

The Caesar Salad

Preparation Time: 10 minutes
Cooking Time: 10 minutes
Total time: 20 minutes
Serves 4 to 6 people

Ingredients

- 1/2 cup bread cubes
- Drizzling extra-virgin olive oil
- 2 bunches chopped romaine lettuce
- Caesar Dressing from scratch*
- 2 thinly sliced radishes

- 11/2 cup roasted chickpeas
- 1/3 cup shaved Pecorino or Parmesan
- 2 tablespoons chives, chopped
- 2 tbsp. toasted pine nuts
- freshly sea salt and ground black pepper

Directions:

1. Preheat the oven to 350 degrees Fahrenheit and line a baking sheet with parchment paper.
2. Prepare the croutons. Toss the bread cubes with olive oil and salt on a baking sheet and bake for 10 minutes, or until toasted.
3. Place the romaine on a platter. Drizzle half of the dressing over the salad, then top with the radishes, croutons, and chickpeas and drizzle with the remaining dressing.
4. Serve with the pecorino, chives, and pine nuts on top. Season to taste with salt and pepper.

The Cobb Salad

Preparation Time: 25 minutes
Cooking Time: 5 minutes
As a side salad, servings: 4

Ingredients:

Ingredients for Chicken Cobb Salad:

- 6 oz bacon, chopped and browned (6 slices)

- 5 cups chopped, rinsed, and dried romaine lettuce from 1 medium head
- 2 cooked chicken breasts
- 2 eggs, hard-boiled
- 1 large sliced avocado
- 1 cup halved cherry tomatoes
- 1/2 cup thinly sliced red onion
- 1/2 cup crumbled blue cheese (or feta cheese)
- 2 tbsp finely chopped parsley

Dressing for a Cobb Salad:

- 3 tablespoons balsamic vinegar
- 1 tablespoon Dijon mustard
- 1 garlic clove, minced or pressed
- 1/3 cup virgin olive oil
- 1/4 teaspoon salt
- 1/8 teaspoon black pepper

Directions:

1. Cook chopped bacon in a skillet until browned and crisp (5 minutes), then transfer to a plate lined with paper towels to cool. Peel and quarter two hard-boiled eggs.
2. Chop, rinse, and spin dry the romaine lettuce before arranging it on a platter. Arrange the remaining salad ingredients (chicken, eggs, avocado, tomatoes, onion,

blue cheese, and bacon) in rows on top of the salad, then sprinkle with the finely chopped parsley.

3. Shake the dressing ingredients in a mason jar vigorously. Drizzle dressing over salad right before serving, or allow guests to add their own dressing to taste.

Greek Salad

Preparation Time: 15 minutes
Total Time: 15 minutes and 15 seconds
As a side salad, servings: 6

Ingredients:

Ingredients for Greek Salad:

- 1 chopped romaine lettuce head
- 1/2 medium thinly sliced red onion
- 1/2 chopped bell pepper (any color)
- 1 cup halved cherry or grape tomatoes (or sliced heirlooms when in season)
- 1 sliced English cucumber
- 1 peeled, pitted, and sliced avocado
- 1/2 cup kalamata olives, cut in thirds
- 4 oz crumbled feta cheese

Ingredients for Greek Dressing:

- 3 tablespoons extra virgin olive oil
- 3 tablespoons lemon juice (from one large lemon)
- 1 garlic clove, minced or pressed
- 1/2 teaspoon sea salt

- 1/4 teaspoon black pepper

Directions:

1. Rinse, chop, and spin dry the romaine lettuce before placing it in a large salad bowl.
2. In the bowl, combine the remaining salad ingredients: sliced red onion, sliced bell peppers, halved tomatoes, diced cucumber, diced avocado, kalamata olives, and feta cheese.
3. Shake together all of the Greek dressing ingredients in a mason jar. Drizzle dressing over salad and toss to combine just before serving.

Garden Salad

Preparation time: 10 minutes
Cooking time: 5 minutes
Total time: 15 minutes and 15 seconds

Ingredients:

For the ranch dressing:

- 1 tablespoon buttermilk
- 1 tablespoon mayonnaise
- 6 tbsp soured cream
- 1 tablespoon minced red onion
- 1 tablespoon minced fresh dill
- 1 tablespoon minced fresh parsley

- 1 minced garlic clove
- 1 teaspoon freshly squeezed lemon juice
- 1 tsp sugar
- freshly ground black pepper and salt

To make the salad:

- 8 cups romaine, green leaf, or iceberg lettuce, torn into bite-sized pieces (see note 2)
- 1 cored and chopped blub endive (see note 3)
- 1-pint grape tomatoes, cut in half lengthwise (see note 4)
- 4 radishes, trimmed at the ends, halved lengthwise and sliced
- 2 peeled, halved lengthwise, and sliced carrots
- 2 Persian cucumbers or 1 hothouse cucumber, cut in half lengthwise

Directions:

1. In a medium mixing bowl, combine buttermilk, mayonnaise, sour cream, red onion, dill, parsley, garlic, lemon juice, sugar, and salt and pepper to taste (I like 1/2 teaspoon salt and 1/4 teaspoon pepper). Refrigerate for at least 10 minutes to allow flavors to blend. Before serving, whisk to recombine.
2. To make the salad, combine lettuce, endive, tomatoes, radishes, carrots, and cucumbers in a large mixing bowl. Drizzle with salad dressing and toss to coat evenly.

Quinoa Salad

Preparation time: 10 minutes
Total time: 10 minutes
Servings:6

Ingredients:

To make the dressing:

- 1 tablespoon olive oil
- 1 minced garlic clove
- 1 large lemon, 2 tablespoons lemon juice
- 1 tablespoon golden balsamic or champagne vinegar
- 1 tsp pure maple syrup (or honey)
- To taste, kosher salt and black pepper

Salad Ingredients:

- 2 cups quinoa, cold cooked
- 2 cups chopped fresh spinach leaves
- 1 cup cucumber, chopped
- 1 cup grape or cherry tomatoes, halved
- 1 large pitted, peeled, and chopped avocado
- 2 sliced green onions
- To taste, kosher salt and black pepper

Directions:

1. Make the dressing first. In a small bowl or jar, combine the olive oil, garlic, lemon juice, vinegar, maple syrup or honey, salt, and pepper. Place aside.
2. Combine the quinoa, spinach, cucumber, tomatoes, avocado, and green onions in a large mixing bowl.

3. Drizzle dressing over the salad and gently stir until it is evenly coated. Season to taste with salt and pepper. Serve.

Black Bean Salad

Preparation time: 15 minutes
Total time: 15 minutes
Servings:6

Ingredients

- 15 oz rinsed and drained can of black beans
- 1 cup corn, 1 large ear sweet corn, or 1 cup frozen corn defrosted
- 1 cup cherry or grape tomatoes, halved
- 1 cup red bell pepper, chopped
- 1/2 cup red onion, chopped
- 1/2 cup cilantro, chopped
- 1 1/2 lime juice
- 1 teaspoon olive oil
- 1 tsp. kosher salt
- 1/2 tsp chili powder
- 1/4 teaspoon cumin powder
- 1 large pitted, peeled, and chopped avocado

Directions:

1. Combine black beans, corn, tomatoes, red pepper, onion, cilantro, lime juice, olive oil, salt, chili powder, and cumin in a large mixing bowl. To combine, stir everything together.

2. Gently fold in the avocado and season with salt, if desired. Serve.

Mango Salsa

Preparation Time: 15 minutes
Time allotted: 15 minutes
Servies 3 cups

Ingredients:

- 3 diced ripe mangos (see photos)
- 1 medium chopped red bell pepper
- 1/2 cup red onion, chopped
- 1/4 cup chopped packed fresh cilantro leaves
- 1 seeded and minced jalapeo
- 1 large lime
- salt, to taste

Directions:

1. Combine the mango, bell pepper, onion, cilantro, and jalapeo in a serving bowl. Drizzle with one lime juice.
2. Stir the ingredients together with a large spoon. Season with salt to taste, and stir once more. Allow the salsa to rest for 10 minutes or more for the best flavor.

There is a community of people who can relate to what you're going through, so you're not alone in this.

Chapter 5:
Vegetarian

Lentil Tacos

Preparation time: 10 minutes
Cooking time: 40 minutes
Total time: 50 minutes
Servings per recipe: 6 tacos

Ingredients:

- 1 cup uncooked lentils
- 4 teaspoons dried minced onion (or onion powder)
- 3 teaspoons chili powder
- 1 teaspoon garlic powder
- 1/2 teaspoon salt
- 1/2 teaspoon paprika
- 1 teaspoon ground cumin
- 1/8 - 1/4 teaspoons cayenne pepper (use more or less depending on your heat preference)
- 1/2 teaspoon dried oregano
- 1/2 teaspoon dried oregano

Directions:

1. In a mixing bowl, combine dried minced onion (or onion powder), chili powder, garlic powder, salt, paprika, cumin, cayenne pepper, and oregano.

2. Sauté onion, garlic, and bell pepper in a large pan (with a lid) over medium-high heat for 3 to 5 minutes.
3. Stir in the lentils and seasoning mix. Cook for 5 minutes.
4. Bring the veggie broth to a boil.
5. Once boiling, cover and reduce heat to low. Cook for 30 minutes, or until the broth has been absorbed and the lentils have softened but are not mushy.
6. Transfer lentils to a bowl and mash with a fork.
7. Warm the tortillas on a skilled or bake them in the oven to make taco shells. Top with tomatoes, avocado, lettuce, and salsa in tortillas.

Tofu Scramble

15 minutes total.
Servings:2
30 minutes total time

Ingredients:

- 1 block extra firm tofu, pressed and crumbled
- 1/2 onion, chopped
- 1 green bell pepper, chopped
- 1/4 cup chopped fresh cilantro
- 1 teaspoon olive oil
- 1/4 teaspoon black pepper
- 1/4 teaspoon salt

Directions:

1. In a medium skillet over medium heat, heat the olive oil. Cook until the onion and bell pepper are softened, about 5 minutes.
2. Cook, stirring frequently, until the tofu is heated through, about 5 minutes more.
3. Combine the cilantro, pepper, and salt in a mixing bowl. Serve right away.

Portobello Mushroom Burger

Two Servings

Ingredients:

- 2 portobello mushrooms, trimmed
- 1 tablespoon extra-virgin olive oil
- 1/4 teaspoon black pepper 1/2 teaspoon salt
- 1/4 cup red onion, chopped
- 1/4 cup fresh cilantro, chopped
- 1/4 sliced avocado
- 2 hamburger buns made from whole wheat

Directions:

1. Preheat the oven to 400° Fahrenheit.
2. Season the portobello mushrooms with salt and pepper after brushing them with olive oil. Bake for 15 minutes, or until tender, on a baking sheet.

3. Heat a small skillet over medium heat while the mushrooms bake. Cook until the onion is softened, about 5 minutes. Add the cilantro and mix well.
4. Place a portobello mushroom on each hamburger bun to assemble the burgers. Avocado slices and onion-cilantro mixture on top. Serve right away.

Quinoa Salad with Roasted Vegetables

1 hour and 15 minutes total time
Four Servings

Ingredients:

- 1 quinoa cup
- 2 tbsp of olive oil
- 1/4 teaspoon black pepper 1/2 teaspoon salt
- 1 broccoli head, cut into florets
- 1 chopped red onion
- 1 diced sweet potato
- 1/4 cup fresh parsley, chopped

Directions:

1. Preheat the oven to 400° Fahrenheit.
2. Toss the broccoli, onion, and sweet potato in a bowl with the olive oil, salt, and pepper. Roast for 30 minutes, or until tender, on a baking sheet.
3. Cook the quinoa according to package directions while the vegetables roast.

4. Allow the quinoa to cool slightly after it has been cooked. Stir in the roasted vegetables and parsley to combine. Serve right away.

Lentil Soup with Whole-Wheat Bread

1 hour and 30 minutes total time
Six Servings

Ingredients:

- 1-pound red lentils
- 2 cups veggie broth
- 1 onion, diced 2 carrots
- Diced 2 celery stalks
- 1 teaspoon garlic powder
- a half teaspoon of dried thyme
- 1/4 teaspoon ground black pepper
- a quarter teaspoon of salt
- 1 tablespoon lemon juice

Directions:

1. In a fine mesh strainer, rinse the lentils.
2. Combine the lentils, vegetable broth, onion, carrots, celery, garlic powder, thyme, pepper, and salt in a large pot. Bring to a boil, then reduce to low heat and continue to cook for 30 minutes, or until the lentils are tender.
3. Serve with whole-wheat bread after adding the lemon juice.

Vegetable Stir-Fry with Brown Rice

30 minutes total time
Four Servings

Ingredients:

- 1 tablespoon extra-virgin olive oil
- 1 onion, chopped
- 2 garlic cloves, minced
- 1 green bell pepper, chopped
- 1 red bell pepper, chopped
- 1 broccoli floret, chopped
- 1/2 cup fresh cilantro, chopped
- 1/4 teaspoon ground black pepper
- a quarter teaspoon of salt
- 2 cups brown rice, cooked

Directions:

1. In a large skillet or wok, heat the olive oil over medium heat. Cook until the onion and garlic are softened, about 5 minutes.
2. Cook until the bell peppers and broccoli are tender, about 7 minutes more.
3. Combine the cilantro, pepper, and salt in a mixing bowl. Serve right away over brown rice.

Tofu Pad Thai with Whole-Wheat Noodles

30 minutes total time
Four Servings

Ingredients:

- 1 extra firm tofu block, pressed and diced
- 1 tablespoon extra virgin olive oil
- 1 chopped onion 2 minced garlic cloves
- 1 chopped red bell pepper 1 chopped green bell pepper
- 1/2 cup fresh cilantro, chopped
- 1 tablespoon tamari sauce
- 1 tablespoon rice vinegar
- 1 tablespoon coconut milk
- 1 teaspoon of brown sugar
- 1/2 teaspoon ground black pepper
- 1 pound whole-wheat noodles 1/4 teaspoon salt

Directions:

1. In a large skillet or wok, heat the olive oil over medium heat. Cook until the tofu is browned on all sides, about 5 minutes.
2. Cook until the onion, garlic, and bell peppers are softened, about 7 minutes more.
3. Combine the cilantro, tamari sauce, rice vinegar, coconut milk, brown sugar, pepper, and salt in a mixing bowl. Return to a simmer and cook for another 2 minutes.
4. In the meantime, prepare the whole-wheat noodles according to package directions.

5. Drain the noodles and combine them with the tofu and sauce in the skillet. Toss everything together and serve right away.

Making Acid Reflux-Friendly Tofu Pad Thai:

- Instead of traditional rice noodles, try whole-wheat noodles. Whole-wheat noodles are easier to digest and are less likely to cause acid reflux symptoms.
- Instead of peanut butter, use coconut milk. Coconut milk contains more healthy fats than peanut butter and is less likely to upset your stomach.
- Instead of soy sauce, use tamari sauce. Tamari sauce is a low-sodium soy sauce that is less likely to cause acid reflux symptoms.
- Chili peppers and other spicy ingredients should be avoided. Spicy foods can irritate your stomach and cause acid reflux.

Vegetarian Lentil Soup

Total time:1hour
Six servings

Ingredients:

- 1 pound red lentils
- 2 cups veggie broth
- 1 onion, diced 2 carrots
- diced 2 celery stalks
- 1 teaspoon garlic powder
- a half teaspoon of dried thyme

- 1/4 teaspoon ground black pepper
- a quarter teaspoon of salt
- 1 tablespoon lemon juice

Directions:

1. In a fine mesh strainer, rinse the lentils.
2. Combine the lentils, vegetable broth, onion, carrots, celery, garlic powder, thyme, pepper, and salt in a large pot. Bring to a boil, then reduce to low heat and continue to cook for 30 minutes, or until the lentils are tender.
3. Serve with whole-wheat bread after adding the lemon juice.

Chapter 6:
Poultry and Seafood

Grilled Salmon with Roasted Vegetables

Total time spent: 30 minutes
Four Servings

Ingredients:

- 4 salmon fillets (each 6 ounces)
- 1 tablespoon extra virgin olive oil
- 1 teaspoon of salt
- 1/4 teaspoon ground black pepper
- 1 cup chopped vegetables (broccoli, Brussels sprouts, zucchini, carrots, etc.)

Directions:

1. Heat the grill to medium-high.
2. Season the salmon fillets with salt and pepper after brushing them with olive oil.
3. Grill the salmon fillets for 6-8 minutes on each side, or until done.
4. While the salmon is grilling, roast the vegetables in a 400°F preheated oven for 15-20 minutes, or until tender.
5. With roasted vegetables, serve the salmon fillets.

Chicken Stir-Fry with Brown Rice

Ingredients:

- 1 tablespoon extra virgin olive oil
- 1 pound boneless, skinless chicken breasts, sliced
- 1 chopped onion
- 2 minced garlic cloves
- 1 chopped green bell pepper
- 1 chopped red bell pepper
- 1/2 cup broccoli florets, chopped
- 1/4 cup soy sauce (low sodium)
- 1 tablespoon rice vinegar
- 1 teaspoon cornstarch
- 1/4 teaspoon ground black pepper
- a quarter teaspoon of salt
- 2 cups brown rice, cooked

Directions:

1. In a large skillet or wok, heat the olive oil over medium-high heat.
2. Cook until the chicken is browned on all sides.
3. Cook until the onion, garlic, bell peppers, and broccoli are softened, about 5 minutes.
4. Whisk together the soy sauce, rice vinegar, cornstarch, pepper, and salt in a small bowl. Cook until the sauce has thickened, about 1 minute, in the skillet with the chicken and vegetables.

5. Serve right away over brown rice.

Shrimp Scampi with Whole-Wheat Pasta

Total time spent: 20 minutes
Four Servings

Ingredients:

- 1 tablespoon extra virgin olive oil
- 1 pound peeled and deveined shrimp
- 1/4 cup white wine
- 1 tablespoon lemon juice
- 1/4 cup fresh chopped parsley
- 1/4 teaspoon garlic powder
- 1/4 teaspoon ground black pepper
- 1 pound whole-wheat pasta 1/4 teaspoon salt

Directions:

1. Prepare the pasta according to the package directions.
2. In a large skillet over medium heat, heat the olive oil while the pasta is cooking.
3. Cook until the shrimp are pink and cooked through, about 2-3 minutes per side.
4. To the skillet, add the white wine, lemon juice, parsley, garlic powder, pepper, and salt. Bring to a simmer and cook for 1-2 minutes, or until the sauce is slightly thickened.
5. Drain the pasta and combine it with the shrimp and sauce in the skillet. Toss everything together and serve right away.

Roasted Chicken with Potatoes and Carrots

1 hour, 30 minutes total time
Six Servings

Ingredients:

- 1 whole (3-4 pound) chicken
- 1 tablespoon extra virgin olive oil
- 1/4 teaspoon black pepper
- 1/2 teaspoon salt
- 1 pound peeled and cut into bite-sized pieces of potatoes
- 1 pound peeled and cut carrots into bite-sized pieces

Directions:

1. Preheat the oven to 400° Fahrenheit.
2. Season the chicken with salt and pepper after rubbing it with olive oil.
3. Arrange the potatoes and carrots around the chicken in a roasting pan.
4. 1 hour and 15 minutes, or until the chicken is cooked through and the vegetables are tender, roast the chicken and vegetables.
5. Allow 10 minutes for the chicken to rest before carving and serving.

Lemon-herb salmon with Roasted Vegetables

Ingredients:

- 4 salmon fillets (each 6 ounces)
- 1 tablespoon extra virgin olive oil
- 1/4 teaspoon black pepper
- 1/4 teaspoon salt
- 1 tsp. dried oregano
- a half teaspoon of dried thyme
- 1 tablespoon lemon juice
- 1 cup chopped vegetables (broccoli, Brussels sprouts, zucchini, carrots, etc.)

Directions:

1. Preheat the oven to 400° Fahrenheit.
2. Season the salmon fillets with salt, pepper, oregano, and thyme after brushing them with olive oil.
3. Line a baking sheet with parchment paper and place the salmon fillets on it.
4. Cook the salmon fillets for 12-15 minutes, or until done.
5. While the salmon is roasting, roast the vegetables in a 400°F preheated oven for 15-20 minutes, or until tender.
6. Salmon fillets should be served with roasted vegetables and lemon juice.

···

Keep moving, you will surely get to your healing point!

···

Chapter 7:
Desserts

Fresh Fruit Salad

Ingredients:

- 1 cup fresh blueberries
- 1 cup hulled and quartered strawberries
- 1 cup fresh raspberries
- 1/2 cup grapes, chopped
- 1 tablespoon lemon juice
- 1 tablespoon honey

Directions:

1. Combine the blueberries, strawberries, raspberries, and grapes in a large mixing bowl.
2. Whisk together the lemon juice and honey in a small bowl.
3. Toss the fruit with the lemon juice and honey mixture to combine.
4. Serve right away or chill for later.

Angel Food Cake with Berries

Ingredients:

- 1.5 cup cake flour
- 12 large room temperature egg whites
- 1 1/4 cup of granulated sugar
- 1 tablespoon cream of tartar
- 1 teaspoon vanilla extract
- 1/4 teaspoon salt
- 1 cup fresh berries (blueberries, strawberries, raspberries, etc.)

Directions:

1. Preheat the oven to 375°F (190°C).
2. In a medium mixing bowl, sift together cake flour and granulated sugar.
3. In a large mixing bowl, whisk together the egg whites, cream of tartar, and salt until stiff peaks form.
4. Fold in the flour mixture gently until just combined.
5. Mix in the vanilla extract.
6. Pour the batter into a 10-inch ungreased tube pan.
7. Bake the cake for 30-35 minutes, or until a toothpick inserted into the center comes out clean.
8. Before serving, allow the cake to cool completely.
9. To serve, cut the cake into slices and top with fresh berries.

Baked Apples with Cinnamon and Honey

Total time required: 45 minutes
Four Servings

Ingredients:

- 4 cored and halved apples
- 1 tablespoon honey
- 1 teaspoon cinnamon powder

Directions:

1. Preheat the oven to 375°F (190°C).
2. In a baking dish, place the apple halves.
3. Drizzle with honey and sprinkle with cinnamon over the apples.
4. Bake the apples for 30-35 minutes, or until tender.
5. Serve right away or chill for later.

Whole-wheat flour and Oats Cookies

Total time spent: 30 minutes
Twelve Servings

Ingredients:

- 1 cup whole-grain flour
- 1 cup rolled oats
- 1 tsp. baking powder
- a half teaspoon baking soda
- 1/4 teaspoon salt
- 1/4 teaspoon cinnamon powder
- 1/4 cup softened butter
- 1 pound brown sugar

- 1 tablespoon granulated sugar
- 1 egg
- a tsp vanilla extract

Directions:

1. Preheat oven to 350°F/175°C.
2. Line a baking sheet with parchment paper.
3. Whisk together the flour, oats, baking powder, baking soda, salt, and cinnamon in a medium mixing bowl.
4. Cream together the butter, brown sugar, and granulated sugar in a large mixing bowl until light and fluffy.
5. Incorporate the egg and vanilla extract.
6. Mix the dry ingredients with the wet ingredients until just combined.
7. Drop the dough onto the prepared baking sheet in rounded tablespoons.
8. Bake the cookies for 10-12 minutes, or until golden brown.
9. Allow the cookies to cool on the baking sheet for a few minutes before transferring to a wire rack to cool completely.

Chapter 8:
Sauces and Broths

Alfredo Sauce

Total time spent: 15 minutes
Four Servings

Ingredients:

- 1 tablespoon extra-virgin olive oil
- 1 tablespoon all-purpose flour
- 2 quarts milk
- 1/4 teaspoon salt
- 1/2 cup grated Parmesan cheese
- 1/4 teaspoon ground black pepper

Directions:

1. In a medium saucepan over medium heat, heat the olive oil.
2. Whisk in the flour until smooth.
3. Whisk in the milk gradually until the sauce is smooth and thickens.
4. Remove from the heat and add the Parmesan cheese, salt, and pepper to taste.
5. Serve right away with pasta or vegetables.

Pesto Sauce

Total time spent: 10 minutes
Four Servings

Ingredients:

- 1 cup basil leaves, fresh
- 1/4 cup pine nuts
- 2 minced garlic cloves
- 1/2 cup Parmesan cheese, grated
- 1 tablespoon olive oil
- 1/4 teaspoon black pepper
- 1/4 teaspoon salt

Directions:

1. Combine the basil leaves, pine nuts, garlic, Parmesan cheese, olive oil, salt, and pepper in a food processor.
2. Blend until smooth.
3. Serve right away with pasta or vegetables.

Vegetable Broth

1 hour is the total time.
Six Servings

Ingredients:

- 1 onion
- diced 2 carrots
- diced 2 celery stalks
- diced 1 teaspoon garlic powder
- 1 teaspoon thyme dried

- 1/2 teaspoon ground black pepper
- 8 c. water

Directions:

1. Combine the onion, carrots, celery, garlic powder, thyme, and pepper in a large pot.
2. Bring to a boil with the water.
3. Reduce the heat to low and continue to cook for 1 hour.
4. Remove the vegetables and strain the broth.

The Chicken Broth

1 hour is the total time.
Six Servings

Ingredients:

1 whole (3-4 pound) chicken

1 onion

diced 2 carrots

diced 2 celery stalks

diced 1 teaspoon garlic powder

1 teaspoon thyme dried

1/2 teaspoon ground black pepper

8 c. water

Directions:

1. Combine the chicken, onion, carrots, celery, garlic powder, thyme, pepper, and water in a large pot.
2. Bring to a boil, then reduce to low heat and cook for 1 hour.
3. Remove the chicken from the pot and set it aside to cool.
4. Remove the bones from the chicken and shred the meat.
5. Serve the chicken meat back in the pot.

20-Week Meal Planner

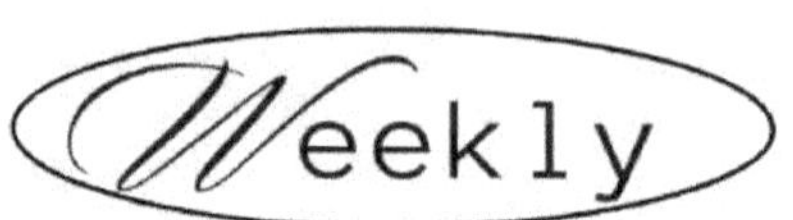

MEAL PLANNER

WEEK __________________

MONTH __________________

MONDAY
BREAKFAST:

LUNCH:

DINNER:

SNACK:

TUESDAY
BREAKFAST:

LUNCH:

DINNER:

SNACK:

WEDNESDAY
BREAKFAST:

LUNCH:

DINNER:

SNACK:

THURSDAY
BREAKFAST:

LUNCH:

DINNER:

SNACK:

FRIDAY
BREAKFAST:

LUNCH:

DINNER:

SNACK:

SATURDAY
BREAKFAST:

LUNCH:

DINNER:

SNACK:

SUNDAY
BREAKFAST:

LUNCH:

DINNER:

SNACK:

NOTES

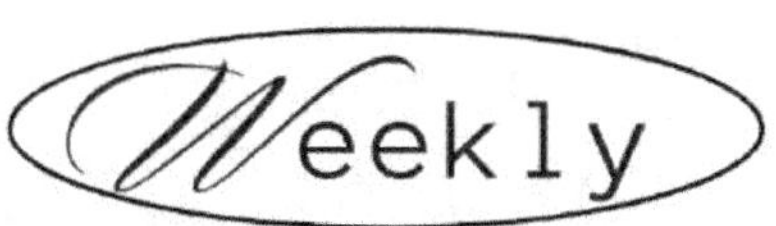

MEAL PLANNER

WEEK _______________   **MONTH** _______________

MONDAY
BREAKFAST:

LUNCH:

DINNER:

SNACK:

TUESDAY
BREAKFAST:

LUNCH:

DINNER:

SNACK:

WEDNESDAY
BREAKFAST:

LUNCH:

DINNER:

SNACK:

THURSDAY
BREAKFAST:

LUNCH:

DINNER:

SNACK:

FRIDAY
BREAKFAST:

LUNCH:

DINNER:

SNACK:

SATURDAY
BREAKFAST:

LUNCH:

DINNER:

SNACK:

SUNDAY
BREAKFAST:

LUNCH:

DINNER:

SNACK:

NOTES

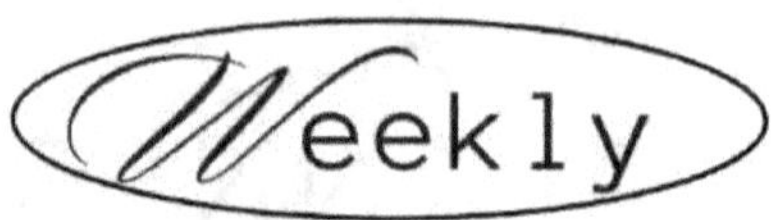 Weekly MEAL PLANNER

WEEK _______________________   **MONTH** _______________________

MONDAY
BREAKFAST:

LUNCH:

DINNER:

SNACK:

TUESDAY
BREAKFAST:

LUNCH:

DINNER:

SNACK:

WEDNESDAY
BREAKFAST:

LUNCH:

DINNER:

SNACK:

THURSDAY
BREAKFAST:

LUNCH:

DINNER:

SNACK:

FRIDAY
BREAKFAST:

LUNCH:

DINNER:

SNACK:

SATURDAY
BREAKFAST:

LUNCH:

DINNER:

SNACK:

SUNDAY
BREAKFAST:

LUNCH:

DINNER:

SNACK:

NOTES

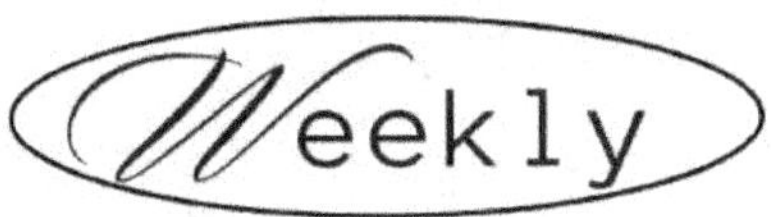

MEAL PLANNER

WEEK _______________________   **MONTH** _______________________

MONDAY
BREAKFAST:

LUNCH:

DINNER:

SNACK:

TUESDAY
BREAKFAST:

LUNCH:

DINNER:

SNACK:

WEDNESDAY
BREAKFAST:

LUNCH:

DINNER:

SNACK:

THURSDAY
BREAKFAST:

LUNCH:

DINNER:

SNACK:

FRIDAY
BREAKFAST:

LUNCH:

DINNER:

SNACK:

SATURDAY
BREAKFAST:

LUNCH:

DINNER:

SNACK:

SUNDAY
BREAKFAST:

LUNCH:

DINNER:

SNACK:

NOTES

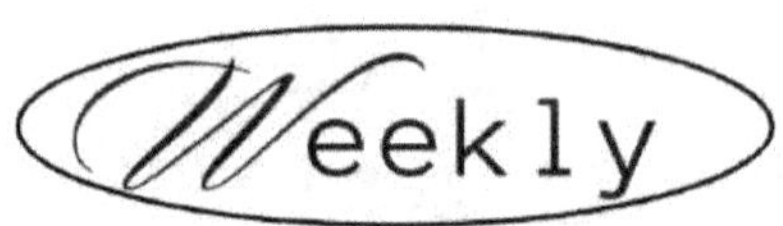

MEAL PLANNER

WEEK ______________________   MONTH ______________________

MONDAY
BREAKFAST:

LUNCH:

DINNER:

SNACK:

TUESDAY
BREAKFAST:

LUNCH:

DINNER:

SNACK:

WEDNESDAY
BREAKFAST:

LUNCH:

DINNER:

SNACK:

THURSDAY
BREAKFAST:

LUNCH:

DINNER:

SNACK:

FRIDAY
BREAKFAST:

LUNCH:

DINNER:

SNACK:

SATURDAY
BREAKFAST:

LUNCH:

DINNER:

SNACK:

SUNDAY
BREAKFAST:

LUNCH:

DINNER:

SNACK:

NOTES

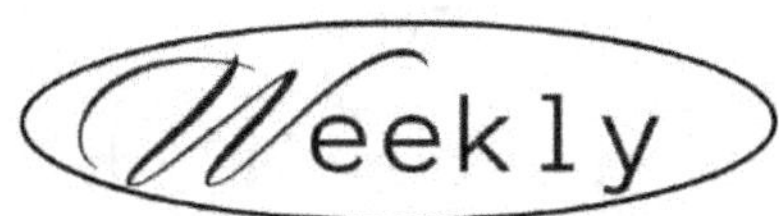

Weekly

MEAL PLANNER

WEEK ___________________________   **MONTH** ___________________________

MONDAY
BREAKFAST:

LUNCH:

DINNER:

SNACK:

TUESDAY
BREAKFAST:

LUNCH:

DINNER:

SNACK:

WEDNESDAY
BREAKFAST:

LUNCH:

DINNER:

SNACK:

THURSDAY
BREAKFAST:

LUNCH:

DINNER:

SNACK:

FRIDAY
BREAKFAST:

LUNCH:

DINNER:

SNACK:

SATURDAY
BREAKFAST:

LUNCH:

DINNER:

SNACK:

SUNDAY
BREAKFAST:

LUNCH:

DINNER:

SNACK:

NOTES

MEAL PLANNER

WEEK _______________________   **MONTH** _______________________

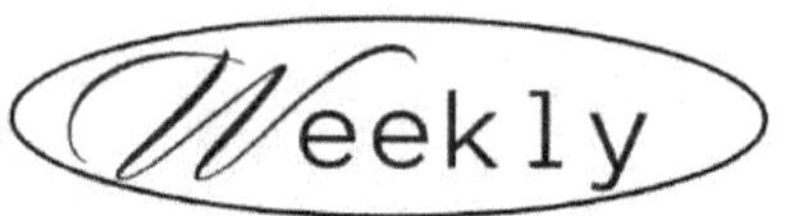

MONDAY
BREAKFAST:

LUNCH:

DINNER:

SNACK:

TUESDAY
BREAKFAST:

LUNCH:

DINNER:

SNACK:

WEDNESDAY
BREAKFAST:

LUNCH:

DINNER:

SNACK:

THURSDAY
BREAKFAST:

LUNCH:

DINNER:

SNACK:

FRIDAY
BREAKFAST:

LUNCH:

DINNER:

SNACK:

SATURDAY
BREAKFAST:

LUNCH:

DINNER:

SNACK:

SUNDAY
BREAKFAST:

LUNCH:

DINNER:

SNACK:

NOTES

○ _______________________
○ _______________________
○ _______________________
○ _______________________
○ _______________________
○ _______________________
○ _______________________
○ _______________________
○ _______________________
○ _______________________
○ _______________________
○ _______________________
○ _______________________

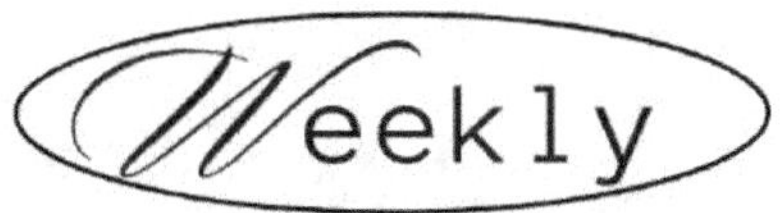

MEAL PLANNER

WEEK _______________   **MONTH** _______________

MONDAY
BREAKFAST:

LUNCH:

DINNER:

SNACK:

TUESDAY
BREAKFAST:

LUNCH:

DINNER:

SNACK:

WEDNESDAY
BREAKFAST:

LUNCH:

DINNER:

SNACK:

THURSDAY
BREAKFAST:

LUNCH:

DINNER:

SNACK:

FRIDAY
BREAKFAST:

LUNCH:

DINNER:

SNACK:

SATURDAY
BREAKFAST:

LUNCH:

DINNER:

SNACK:

SUNDAY
BREAKFAST:

LUNCH:

DINNER:

SNACK:

NOTES

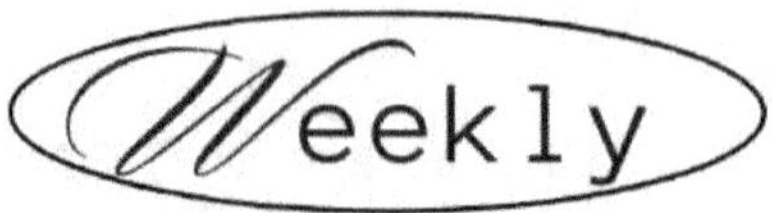

MEAL PLANNER

WEEK _______________________

MONTH _______________________

MONDAY
BREAKFAST:

LUNCH:

DINNER:

SNACK:

TUESDAY
BREAKFAST:

LUNCH:

DINNER:

SNACK:

WEDNESDAY
BREAKFAST:

LUNCH:

DINNER:

SNACK:

THURSDAY
BREAKFAST:

LUNCH:

DINNER:

SNACK:

FRIDAY
BREAKFAST:

LUNCH:

DINNER:

SNACK:

SATURDAY
BREAKFAST:

LUNCH:

DINNER:

SNACK:

SUNDAY
BREAKFAST:

LUNCH:

DINNER:

SNACK:

NOTES

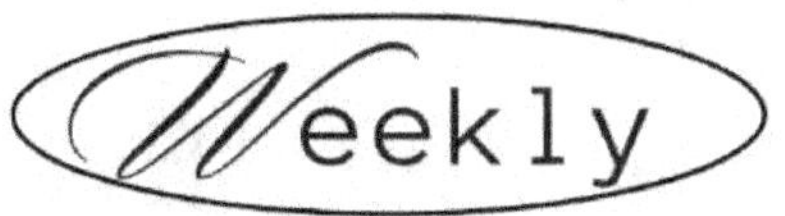

MEAL PLANNER

WEEK _______________   **MONTH** _______________

MONDAY
BREAKFAST:

LUNCH:

DINNER:

SNACK:

TUESDAY
BREAKFAST:

LUNCH:

DINNER:

SNACK:

WEDNESDAY
BREAKFAST:

LUNCH:

DINNER:

SNACK:

THURSDAY
BREAKFAST:

LUNCH:

DINNER:

SNACK:

FRIDAY
BREAKFAST:

LUNCH:

DINNER:

SNACK:

SATURDAY
BREAKFAST:

LUNCH:

DINNER:

SNACK:

SUNDAY
BREAKFAST:

LUNCH:

DINNER:

SNACK:

NOTES

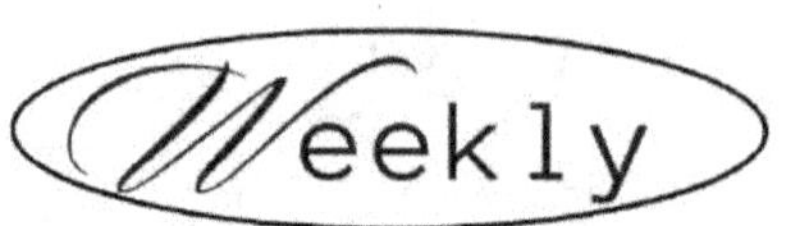

MEAL PLANNER

WEEK ________________________   **MONTH** ________________________

MONDAY
BREAKFAST:

LUNCH:

DINNER:

SNACK:

TUESDAY
BREAKFAST:

LUNCH:

DINNER:

SNACK:

WEDNESDAY
BREAKFAST:

LUNCH:

DINNER:

SNACK:

THURSDAY
BREAKFAST:

LUNCH:

DINNER:

SNACK:

FRIDAY
BREAKFAST:

LUNCH:

DINNER:

SNACK:

SATURDAY
BREAKFAST:

LUNCH:

DINNER:

SNACK:

SUNDAY
BREAKFAST:

LUNCH:

DINNER:

SNACK:

NOTES

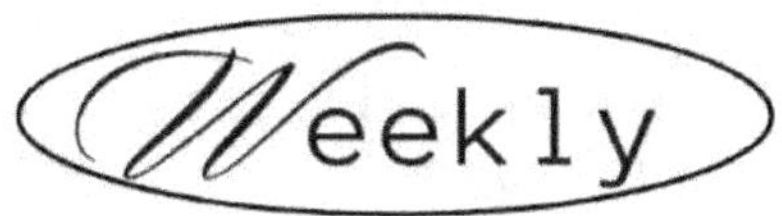

MEAL PLANNER

WEEK _______________________   **MONTH** _______________________

MONDAY
BREAKFAST:

LUNCH:

DINNER:

SNACK:

TUESDAY
BREAKFAST:

LUNCH:

DINNER:

SNACK:

WEDNESDAY
BREAKFAST:

LUNCH:

DINNER:

SNACK:

THURSDAY
BREAKFAST:

LUNCH:

DINNER:

SNACK:

FRIDAY
BREAKFAST:

LUNCH:

DINNER:

SNACK:

SATURDAY
BREAKFAST:

LUNCH:

DINNER:

SNACK:

SUNDAY
BREAKFAST:

LUNCH:

DINNER:

SNACK:

NOTES

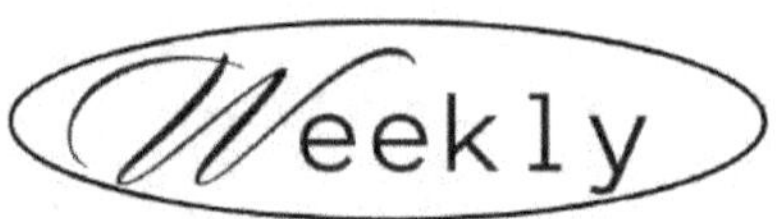

MEAL PLANNER

WEEK ________________________ MONTH ________________________

MONDAY
BREAKFAST:

LUNCH:

DINNER:

SNACK:

TUESDAY
BREAKFAST:

LUNCH:

DINNER:

SNACK:

WEDNESDAY
BREAKFAST:

LUNCH:

DINNER:

SNACK:

THURSDAY
BREAKFAST:

LUNCH:

DINNER:

SNACK:

FRIDAY
BREAKFAST:

LUNCH:

DINNER:

SNACK:

SATURDAY
BREAKFAST:

LUNCH:

DINNER:

SNACK:

SUNDAY
BREAKFAST:

LUNCH:

DINNER:

SNACK:

NOTES

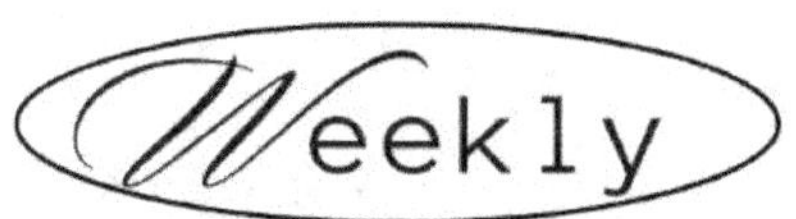

MEAL PLANNER

WEEK _______________________   **MONTH** _______________________

MONDAY
BREAKFAST:

LUNCH:

DINNER:

SNACK:

TUESDAY
BREAKFAST:

LUNCH:

DINNER:

SNACK:

WEDNESDAY
BREAKFAST:

LUNCH:

DINNER:

SNACK:

THURSDAY
BREAKFAST:

LUNCH:

DINNER:

SNACK:

FRIDAY
BREAKFAST:

LUNCH:

DINNER:

SNACK:

SATURDAY
BREAKFAST:

LUNCH:

DINNER:

SNACK:

SUNDAY
BREAKFAST:

LUNCH:

DINNER:

SNACK:

NOTES

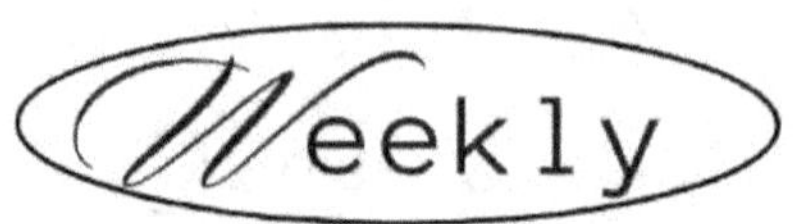

MEAL PLANNER

WEEK _______________________   **MONTH** _______________________

MONDAY
BREAKFAST:

LUNCH:

DINNER:

SNACK:

TUESDAY
BREAKFAST:

LUNCH:

DINNER:

SNACK:

WEDNESDAY
BREAKFAST:

LUNCH:

DINNER:

SNACK:

THURSDAY
BREAKFAST:

LUNCH:

DINNER:

SNACK:

FRIDAY
BREAKFAST:

LUNCH:

DINNER:

SNACK:

SATURDAY
BREAKFAST:

LUNCH:

DINNER:

SNACK:

SUNDAY
BREAKFAST:

LUNCH:

DINNER:

SNACK:

NOTES

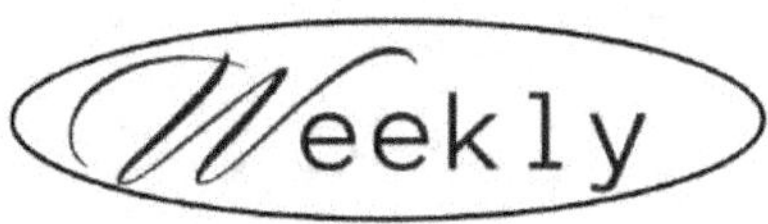

MEAL PLANNER

WEEK _______________________ **MONTH** _______________________

MONDAY
BREAKFAST:

LUNCH:

DINNER:

SNACK:

TUESDAY
BREAKFAST:

LUNCH:

DINNER:

SNACK:

WEDNESDAY
BREAKFAST:

LUNCH:

DINNER:

SNACK:

THURSDAY
BREAKFAST:

LUNCH:

DINNER:

SNACK:

FRIDAY
BREAKFAST:

LUNCH:

DINNER:

SNACK:

SATURDAY
BREAKFAST:

LUNCH:

DINNER:

SNACK:

SUNDAY
BREAKFAST:

LUNCH:

DINNER:

SNACK:

NOTES

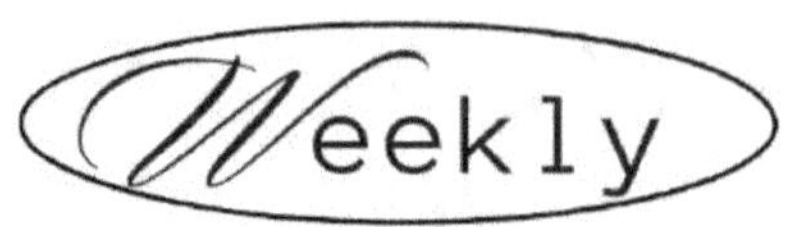

MEAL PLANNER

WEEK _______________________   **MONTH** _______________________

MONDAY
BREAKFAST:

LUNCH:

DINNER:

SNACK:

TUESDAY
BREAKFAST:

LUNCH:

DINNER:

SNACK:

WEDNESDAY
BREAKFAST:

LUNCH:

DINNER:

SNACK:

THURSDAY
BREAKFAST:

LUNCH:

DINNER:

SNACK:

FRIDAY
BREAKFAST:

LUNCH:

DINNER:

SNACK:

SATURDAY
BREAKFAST:

LUNCH:

DINNER:

SNACK:

SUNDAY
BREAKFAST:

LUNCH:

DINNER:

SNACK:

NOTES

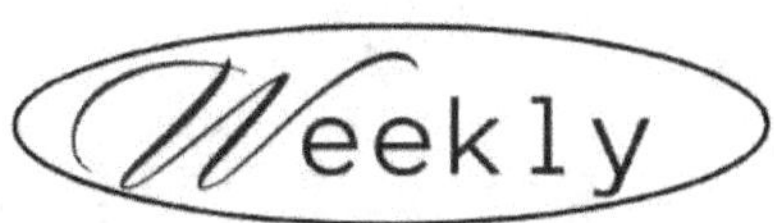

MEAL
PLANNER

WEEK ___________________ **MONTH** ___________________

MONDAY
BREAKFAST:

LUNCH:

DINNER:

SNACK:

TUESDAY
BREAKFAST:

LUNCH:

DINNER:

SNACK:

WEDNESDAY
BREAKFAST:

LUNCH:

DINNER:

SNACK:

THURSDAY
BREAKFAST:

LUNCH:

DINNER:

SNACK:

FRIDAY
BREAKFAST:

LUNCH:

DINNER:

SNACK:

SATURDAY
BREAKFAST:

LUNCH:

DINNER:

SNACK:

SUNDAY
BREAKFAST:

LUNCH:

DINNER:

SNACK:

NOTES

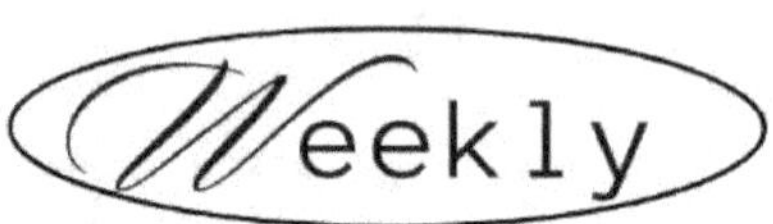

MEAL PLANNER

WEEK ___________________________ **MONTH** ___________________________

MONDAY
BREAKFAST:

LUNCH:

DINNER:

SNACK:

TUESDAY
BREAKFAST:

LUNCH:

DINNER:

SNACK:

WEDNESDAY
BREAKFAST:

LUNCH:

DINNER:

SNACK:

THURSDAY
BREAKFAST:

LUNCH:

DINNER:

SNACK:

FRIDAY
BREAKFAST:

LUNCH:

DINNER:

SNACK:

SATURDAY
BREAKFAST:

LUNCH:

DINNER:

SNACK:

SUNDAY
BREAKFAST:

LUNCH:

DINNER:

SNACK:

NOTES

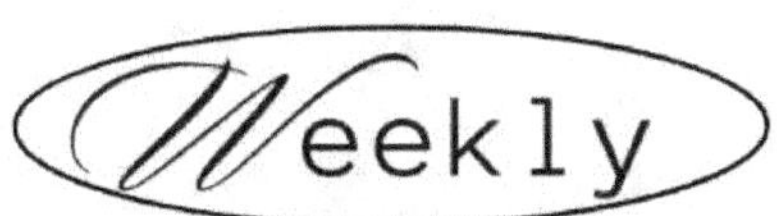

MEAL PLANNER

WEEK __________________________   **MONTH** __________________________

MONDAY
BREAKFAST:

LUNCH:

DINNER:

SNACK:

TUESDAY
BREAKFAST:

LUNCH:

DINNER:

SNACK:

WEDNESDAY
BREAKFAST:

LUNCH:

DINNER:

SNACK:

THURSDAY
BREAKFAST:

LUNCH:

DINNER:

SNACK:

FRIDAY
BREAKFAST:

LUNCH:

DINNER:

SNACK:

SATURDAY
BREAKFAST:

LUNCH:

DINNER:

SNACK:

SUNDAY
BREAKFAST:

LUNCH:

DINNER:

SNACK:

NOTES

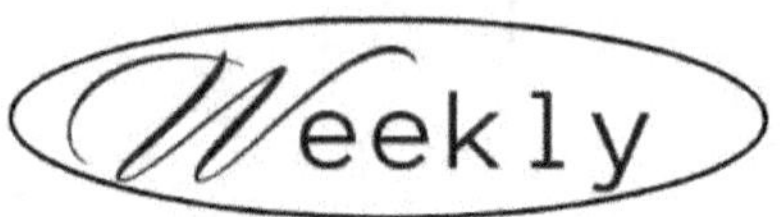

MEAL PLANNER

WEEK ______________________   **MONTH** ______________________

MONDAY
BREAKFAST:

LUNCH:

DINNER:

SNACK:

TUESDAY
BREAKFAST:

LUNCH:

DINNER:

SNACK:

WEDNESDAY
BREAKFAST:

LUNCH:

DINNER:

SNACK:

THURSDAY
BREAKFAST:

LUNCH:

DINNER:

SNACK:

FRIDAY
BREAKFAST:

LUNCH:

DINNER:

SNACK:

SATURDAY
BREAKFAST:

LUNCH:

DINNER:

SNACK:

SUNDAY
BREAKFAST:

LUNCH:

DINNER:

SNACK:

NOTES

Recipes Index

A

B

C

E

F

G

L

Lentil Soup with Whole-Wheat Bread, 47
Lentil Tacos, 43

M

Mango Salsa, 41
Mashed Potatoes, 15
Minestrone Soup, 32

O

Oatmeal with Berries and Nuts, 9

P

Pesto Sauce, 64
Portobello Mushroom Burger, 45

Q

Quinoa Salad, 39
Quinoa Salad with Roasted Vegetables, 46

R

Roasted Chicken with Potatoes and Carrots, 56
Roasted Vegetables, 13

S

Salad with Vinaigrette Dressing, 20
Shrimp Scampi with Whole-Wheat Pasta, 55
Sweet Potato Fries, 17

T

The Caesar Salad, 33
The Chicken Broth, 65
The Cobb Salad, 34
Tofu Pad Thai with Whole-Wheat Noodles, 49

Tofu Scramble, 44
Trail Mix, 25

V

Vegetable Broth, 64
Vegetable Soup, 31
Vegetable Stir-Fry with Brown Rice, 48
Vegetarian Lentil Soup, 50

W

Whole-wheat flour and Oats Cookies, 61
Whole-Wheat Rolls, 18